Juicing Recipes

THE TOP 25 JUICING RECIPES YOU NEED TO GET LEAN, HEALTHY AND FEEL AWESOME!

Introduction

I want to thank you and congratulate you for purchasing the book, *"Juicing recipes: The Top 25 Juicing Recipes You Need to Get Lean, Healthy and Feel Awesome!"*

Do you want to lose weight in a healthy way? Are you too lazy to exercise, yet want to shed some pounds? Well, then you have chosen the right book, as in the course of this book you are about to discover the secret to losing weight and staying fit. You needn't engage in any grueling exercises or go on a stringent diet. All that you will need to do is follow the simple recipes that have been given in this book. You will be pleasantly surprised to find how easily you are able to shed those extra kilos, while drinking these delicious juices. The recipes in this book have incorporated ingredients that are rich in nutrients and dietary fibers that are beneficial for your health.

This book has been tailored to fit the needs of anyone who has health as their goal. The main focus of this book it to provide you with the best juicing recipes that are not only delicious but will also help you in losing weight and staying healthy. It will prove to be the perfect partner for all the dieters who would want to shed a few kilos, while keeping their bodies thoroughly nourished and healthy.

Each recipe also explains the various weight loss benefits the various ingredients used have got to offer so that you can get a better understanding of why a particular fruit or vegetable is good for losing weight and maintain a healthy diet. This book provides the recipes to create healthy juices along with the benefits that each of these recipes has got to offer. The various tips and suggestions regarding mixing different ingredients together will help you in coming up with delicious and healthy recipes that are fun to make. Juices can be teamed up perfectly with any dict that you are on and also the next time you feel like grabbing a sugary snack, you can instead make yourself a delicious and healthy juice by following the recipes that have been given in this book.

If you are tired of feeling lethargic and aren't able to find a suitable weight loss solution that would work for you, then take action immediately and follow the juicing recipes that have been given in this book. This book contains amazing recipes that are easy to follow and make you feel and look awesome.

Thanks again for purchasing this book, I hope you enjoy it!

Table of Contents

Chapter 1: Fruit Juicing Recipes

Fruity Blast

This is a nourishing juice that keeps you pepped up when your energy levels are low. It sweet in taste and changes your mood instantly. The nectarine is the "surprise element" here that has a low glycemic index and will not spike your blood glucose levels.

Did you know: kiwis have high vitamin C content, the highest amongst citrus fruits.

Note: If the pineapple is not ripe, place it upside down to hasten the process of ripening.

The pineapple can be substituted with a ripe papaya. Papaya is low in calories and has tons of vitamins, minerals and phytonutrients.

Ingredients:

- 4 kiwis
- 4 apples
- 2/3 of a small ripe pineapple
- 4 nectarines

Instructions:

1. Peel and chop the kiwis.
2. Core and slice the apples.
3. Deseed the nectarines and chop into pieces.
4. Peel the skin of the pineapple using a sharp knife and chop into pieces.

5. Add all the fruits to the jar of a blender and blend until smooth. If you find the consistency to be very thick, add some water and blend again. Strain using a wire mesh strainer if you desire.

6. Alternately, juice together all the ingredients in a juicer. By blending in a blender, you stand to retain the fiber content of the fruits, while in the juicer; you will miss out the fiber.

7. Pour into glasses. Top with crushed ice and serve.

Health Booster Juice

Pears are great for weight loss as they are rich in fiber. When juiced along with apples and cherries, the resulting concoction is packed with vitamins A, B, C, and E. This juice promotes anti-aging, strengthens bones and gives you a younger looking skin. And., let's face it, who wouldn't like to look younger?

You can substitute the apples with apricots if you prefer. You can also add in some fresh orange pulp for a tangier taste.

Ingredients:

- 2 apples
- 1 cup cherries
- 4 medium ripe and soft pears

Instructions:

1. Core the apples and pears. Chop into large pieces.

2. Pit the cherries.

3. Place all the ingredients in the jar of a blender and blend until smooth. Strain using a wire mesh strainer if you desire. If you find it too thick, dilute it with water.

4. Pour into glasses and serve with ice cubes.

Tropical Berry Blast

Major health benefits come in a small package commonly known as "berries". They are packed with nutrients and are a major source of antioxidants. These antioxidants make your skin healthy, boost your immune system, and make your memory a lot sharper!

You can also add in other berries like blackberries or raspberries into the mix for an enhanced flavor!

Ingredients:

- 1/2 cup blueberries
- 1/2 cup strawberries
- 1 cup mango
- 2 tablespoons water

Instructions:

1. Hull the strawberries and chop them into smaller pieces
2. Peel and deseed the mango and chop into smaller pieces.
3. Add all the ingredients to a blender and blend until smooth. Strain using a wire mesh strainer if you desire. If you find the juice too thick, then dilute it water.
4. Serve with ice cubes topped with a blueberry, a thin slice of mango, and a thin slice of strawberry.

Tangy Apple & Orange Crush

We have often heard the saying, "an apple a day keeps the doctor away", but have we ever pondered why? Well, apples help you to keep your weight in check, detoxify the liver, control cholesterol and are great for your heart. And when combined with some citrus fruits, they are an unstoppable train of nutrition!

Ingredients:

- 2 large oranges
- 1/2 a small pineapple
- 2 medium apples
- 1 lemon
- 2 large peaches

Instructions:

1. Peel the oranges and separate into segments.
2. Peel and chop the pineapples and lemon.
3. Pit the peaches and chop.
4. Core and chop the apples.
5. Place all the ingredients in the blender and blend until smooth. Strain using a wire mesh strainer if you desire. If you find it too thick, dilute it with water. Pour into glasses and serve with ice cubes.

Sweet & Spicy Mango Citrus Juice

What would you do if I told you that the consumption of cayenne pepper aids in the burning of fat? (Please, do not eat more than a dash of that stuff – IT BURNS!) Add a dash of it to your favorite juice – along with burning fat, it will also help in adding a surprisingly good flavor to your boring old juice. Don't believe me? Try it for yourself!

Ingredients:

- 2 mangoes
- 2 apples
- 1 lemon
- 2 large oranges
- 1/8 teaspoon cayenne pepper

Instructions:

1. Peel and deseed the apple. Chop into pieces
2. Peel the oranges and separate into segments.
3. Peel the lemon.
4. Juice the oranges and lemon in a juicer.
5. Add the mango, apple, cayenne pepper and the orange - lemon juice to the jar of a blender and blend until smooth.
6. If you find it too thick, dilute it with water.
7. Pour into glasses and serve with ice cubes.

Apple Cranberry Juice

Cranberries are commonly referred to as "super food"! You can use them to make savory dishes, sauces, desserts and juices due to the versatility of their flavor. But, along with being versatile, they are also extremely healthy! Rich in antioxidants, cranberries have very less calories, lower the risk of UTIs (Urinary Tract Infections), kidney problems, and lower blood pressure and give the immunity system a boost. If that's not super, I don't know what is!

Ingredients:

- 1 cup whole cranberries
- 6 medium apples
- 1 lemon
- 2 inches fresh ginger
- 2 large oranges

Instructions:

1. Core and chop apples into smaller pieces.
2. Peel and slice the ginger
3. Peel the lemon and half it.
4. Peel the orange and separate into segments.
5. Juice the oranges and lemon in a juicer.
6. Add rest of the ingredients to a blender along with the orange and lemon juice.
7. Blend until smooth. If you find it too thick, dilute it with water.
8. Pour into glasses and serve with ice cubes

Chapter 2: Vegetable Juicing Recipes

Low Calorie Vegetable Juice

The Low Cal Vegetable Juice is a fat burner and helps in slimming your waistline. Loaded with fibers and some much-needed Omega- 3, this cooler also has a high satiating quotient. This makes it the ideal "in between meal snack"! Add in a little pepper for a little spicy aftertaste if you wish!

Ingredients:

- 2 cucumbers
- 2 large heads broccoli
- 2 tablespoons lemon juice
- 2 heads romaine lettuce
- 1 cup water

Instructions:

1. Chop the broccoli into smaller florets.
2. Chop the cucumber and lettuce.
3. Add all the ingredients except lemon juice into the jar of a blender and blend until smooth.
4. Strain using a wire mesh strainer if you desire. If you find it too thick, dilute it with water. Pour into glasses. Add lemon juice and stir.
5. Serve with ice cubes.

Tomato, Carrot and Asparagus Juice

This delicious juice helps in the reduction of excessive water retention in the body and suppresses hunger. One glass every day with your regular breakfast ensures that your day begins on a healthy, antioxidant rich note! If you wish for a sweeter flavor in the juice, swipe the carrots for some beetroots – DELICIOUS!

Ingredients:

- 3 large tomatoes
- 6 medium carrots
- 8 stalks asparagus
- 1/2 cup water

Instructions:

1. Chop the tomatoes, carrots and asparagus into smaller pieces.

2. Place all the ingredients in the jar of a blender and blend until smooth. Strain using a wire mesh strainer if you desire. If you find it too thick, dilute it with water.

3. Pour into glasses and serve with ice cubes.

Green Overload

It is known fact that Green = Healthy. Be it due to their high vitamin C content or due to the abundance of fiber, dark green leafy vegetables have become the poster child for healthy foods. So a juice with not one, not two, not three, but FIVE different types of dark green leafy veggies should be named as the health drink of the millennium! With the addition of some carrots, cucumbers and lime juice, this juice tastes delicious and is a great energy booster on those long days when you feel too bored to even move. Go ahead make yourself a glass, I assure you, you won't be disappointed!

Ingredients:

- 1 bunch spinach
- 1 bunch chard
- 1 bunch parsley
- 1 bunch kale
- 1 bunch celery
- 2 cucumbers
- 4 carrots
- 4 tablespoons lime juice

Instructions:

1. Rinse the greens. Drain and set aside.
2. Chop the carrots and cucumbers.
3. Juice together all the ingredients in a juicer.
4. Pour into glasses. Serve with ice cubes.

Immunity Booster Juice

Like the name says, this juice helps in boosting your immune system, ensuring that you stay fit, healthy and disease free! But, bell peppers in a juice, you ask? Bell peppers have a lot of antioxidants and anti-inflammatory properties that ensure you are healthy! Consume one glass of this juice in the morning on an empty stomach and see the wonders it does for your body!

Ingredients:

- 4 bell peppers, any color
- 2 cucumbers
- 2 bunches arugula

Instructions:

1. Rinse and drain arugula.
2. Chop cucumbers.
3. Deseed the bell peppers and chop.
4. Place all the ingredients in the blender and blend until smooth. Strain using a wire mesh strainer if you desire. If you find it too thick, dilute it with water.
5. Pour into glasses and serve with ice cubes.

Cucumber and Celery Juice

This electrolyte rich juice is the ideal post – work out juice – one glass and you will feel refreshed. This is because of the sodium content in the celery and the cooling and hydrating effect of the cucumber present in the juice. Don't like parsley? Add some spinach instead!

Ingredients:

- 12 stalks celery
- 3 medium sized cucumber, chopped
- 1 bunch parsley, chopped
- 2 inch pieces ginger, peeled, sliced
- Juice of a lemon
- A dash of cinnamon

Instructions:

1. Trim and chop the celery and parsley.
2. Peel and slice ginger.
3. Juice all the ingredients in a juicer of blend together in a blender. Sprinkle a dash of cinnamon.
4. Serve over crushed ice.

Watercress and Carrot Juice

Vitamins A & C are two of the most important vitamins required by our body and luckily, this juice has an abundant quantity of both! Skip the fried snacks and make yourself a glass for your evening hunger pangs – you surely won't be disappointed! Switch out the spinach for some Swiss chard if you like it.

Ingredients:

- 6 medium carrots
- 1 cup spinach
- 2 cups watercress
- 4 tomatoes
- Salt and pepper to taste

Instructions:

1. Peel and chop carrots into smaller pieces.
2. Chop the tomatoes into smaller pieces.
3. Rinse and drain spinach and watercress.
4. Juice all the ingredients in a juicer of blend together in a blender. Sprinkle a dash of salt and pepper and stir.
5. Serve with ice.

Chapter 3: Mixing up Fruits and Veggies

By mixing up fruits and vegetables, you get the nutrition and distinctive flavors from both!

Leafy Berry Blast

The leafy berry blast takes the nutritive goodness of the dark green leafy vegetables and the flavor of the berries to give you a drink that is healthy and tasty all at once! This nutrient rich drink is good for your skin and hair and also aids in weight loss. You can add in more berries or more dark green leafy vegetables if you wish to!

Ingredients:

- 3 red apples
- 3 small zucchini
- 6 green or purple kale leaves
- 1 1/2 cup blueberries
- 1 small red cabbage
- 1 small purple or white cauliflower
- 1 medium cucumber
- 2 oranges
- 1/2 cup shredded fresh coconut (to garnish)

Instructions:

1. Trim the cucumber and zucchinis. Chop zucchini and cucumber into smaller pieces.
2. Core the apples and chop into smaller pieces.
3. Peel oranges and separate into segments.

4. Cut cabbage into wedges.

5. Roll the kale leaves.

6. Juice together all the ingredients in a juicer.

7. Pour into glasses. Serve with ice cubes.

Turmeric Sunrise

Turmeric is a well-known spice, used commonly in South East Asia. But, did you know that turmeric has immense medicinal and anti-bacterial properties that "cleanse you from the inside". Combine this with some delicious fruits and vegetables and you have yourself a delicious detox juice!

Ingredients:

- 5 medium carrots
- 3 inches fresh ginger root
- 8 inches fresh turmeric root
- 5 stalks celery
- 3 medium apples
- 3 medium pears
- 3 lemons

Instructions:

1. Peel and chop ginger and turmeric roots.
2. Chop celery into smaller pieces
3. Core the apples and pears. Chop into smaller pieces.
4. Peel the lemons. Halve them. Deseed if necessary.
5. Juice together all the ingredients in a juicer.
6. Pour into glasses. Serve with ice cubes.

Apple and Spinach Detox

The apple and spinach detox is ideal for when you've had a few drinks too many, night after night and your body is a downright mess. Consume this juice daily on an empty stomach for best results.

Ingredients:

- 1 cup lettuce
- 1 cup spinach
- 5 apples
- 1 cucumber
- 2 stalks celery
- Ice as required

Instructions:

1. Peel and chop apples and cucumbers. Peeling the apples and cucumber is optional.
2. Chop celery into smaller pieces.
3. Place all the ingredients in the blender and blend until smooth. Strain using a wire mesh strainer if you desire. If you find it too thick, dilute it with water.
4. Pour into glasses and serve with ice cubes.

Carrot and Grapefruit Juice

Carrots are low on calories and high on fiber, making them the ideal "snack food". But chomping on carrots all day like Bugs Bunny can get a tad bit boring after a while for us non-Bugs Bunny people. Solution? The delicious Carrot and Grapefruit juice loaded with nutrition and immense amount of flavors that will leave your taste buds tingling for more!

Ingredients:

- 6 carrots
- 1 1/2 grapefruits
- 2 inches fresh ginger root
- 4 tablespoons lemon juice

Instructions:

1. Trim and chop the carrots
2. Peel the grapefruit and separate into segments.
3. Peel and slice ginger.
4. Juice together all the ingredients in a juicer.
5. Pour into glasses. Serve with ice cubes.
6. If you want more fiber, then peel and deseed the grapefruit segments. Add all the ingredients to a blender with 1/2-cup water and blend until smooth.

The Veggie Delight

There is nothing better than the Veggie delight to raise your spirits and energy levels after a long tiring day. Containing cabbage, the super food for the brain, this juice can be described to be "good health in a glass". So, what are you waiting for? Go ahead and make yourself a glass!

Ingredients:

- 3 carrots
- 3 oranges
- 2 stalks celery
- 3 large stems of broccoli
- 1/2 head lettuce
- 1/2 small cabbage green or red

Instructions:

1. Chop the carrots and celery.
2. Peel the oranges and separate into segments.
3. Chop the cabbage into wedges.
4. Roll the lettuce leaves.
5. Chop the broccoli into smaller pieces.
6. Juice together all the ingredients in a juicer.
7. Pour into glasses. Serve with ice cubes.

Beet Treat

The beet treat is an ideal pre-workout drink. Not too heavy on the stomach, drinking it just before working out ensures that your body has enough energy to get through the workout with ease! You can add in more berries to add another layer of taste to it!

Ingredients:

- 2 cups strawberries
- 4 beetroots
- 2 red carrots

Instructions:

1. Hull and halve the strawberries
2. Peel and chop the beetroots and carrots.
3. Place all the ingredients in the jar of a blender and blend until smooth. Strain using a wire mesh strainer if you desire. If you find it too thick, dilute it with water. Pour into glasses and serve with ice cubes.

Power Gulp

The Power Gulp is loaded with iron, vitamin K and potassium, making it your easy source of difficult to acquire nutrients. If you wish, add some frozen whole grapes to the juice to chill your juice and add some "crunch" to it!

Ingredients:

- 2 cups seedless green grapes
- 2 small Granny Smith apples
- 2 cups kale
- 2 cucumbers
- 1 cup water

Instructions:

1. Discard hard stem and ribs from kale. Slice the kale.
2. Chop the cucumbers into smaller pieces.
3. Core and chop apples.
4. Place all the ingredients in the blender and blend until smooth. Strain using a wire mesh strainer if you desire. If you find it too thick, dilute it with water. Pour into glasses and serve with ice cubes.
5. Garnish with a slice of cucumber and serve.

Chapter 4: Juicing Heaven: Adding Yogurt to the mix

Probiotics are the healthy bacteria present in foods and the consumption of these probiotics is helpful to your gut and boosts immunity. Juices are great for weight loss and the addition of probiotics to your juice makes the juice healthier. One of the most commonly available probiotic is yogurt.

Various types of yogurts are available in the market today, like plain yogurt, low fat yogurt, full fat yogurt, flavored yogurt, soy yogurt, coconut milk yogurt etc. Once you juice the fruits and vegetables, pour the juice in a bowl of yogurt and stir. If you like it frothy, you can add it while blending. This makes the juice healthier and the yogurt tastier!

Yogurt Mangoloupe

The yogurt Mangoloupe is a tropical and delicious flavored yogurt that has a tangy flavor. A satiating evening snack, the yogurt Mangoloupe has a large amount of vitamin C in it, making it extremely healthy!

Ingredients:

- 10 oranges
- 2 mangoes
- 1 small cantaloupe
- 1/3 cup yogurt

Instructions:

1. Peel and deseed the mango and cantaloupe. Chop into pieces

2. Peel the oranges and separate into segments.

3. Juice together the mangoes, cantaloupe and oranges in a juicer.

4. Add about 3 tablespoons yogurt into 2 bowls.

5. Divide the juice between the bowls. Stir and serve.

Pink Yogurt Smoothie

The pink yogurt smoothie is a vitamin rich drink that tastes out of this world. There is something extremely enticing about the combination of raspberries and yogurt that makes this drink extremely popular with children and adults alike. Add in some red carrots if you wish for a deeper color!

Ingredients:

- 2 apples
- 2 cups raspberries
- 4 oranges
- 2 cups strawberries
- 1 cup plain yogurt

Instructions:

1. Core and chop the apples.
2. Peel the oranges and separate into segments
3. The raspberries and strawberries can be either fresh or frozen.
4. If using fresh strawberries hull the strawberries and halve them.
5. Juice the apples and oranges in a juicer.
6. Add rest of the ingredients to a blender along with the apple-orange juice. Blend until smooth and serve.

Creamy Berry

Berries are loaded with anti-oxidants that help refresh your skin and make it look healthy and glowing. Berries also have an extremely delicious taste and can satisfy the choosiest taste buds. So, the creamy berry is not only healthy, it is also mega delicious!

Ingredients:

- 1 /2 cup raspberries
- 1/2 cup blueberries
- 1/2 cup strawberries
- 1/2 cup blackberries
- 1/2 cup huckleberries
- 1/2 cup cranberries
- 1 cup plain yogurt

Instructions:

1. Hull and halve the strawberries.

2. Add all the ingredients into a blender and blend until smooth.

3. Pour into glasses and serve immediately with crushed ice.

Blackberry Pineapple Smoothie

The blackberry pineapple smoothie is ideal for people who suffer from a high blood pressure issue. The high potassium content in pineapple results in a lowering of blood pressure. You can add in some more berries, such as raspberries or cranberries for added taste.

Ingredients:

- 2 cups pineapple pieces
- 2 cups blackberries
- 1/4 cup water
- 1/3 cup plain yogurt

Instructions:

1. Hull and halve the strawberries.

2. Add all the ingredients into a blender and blend until smooth.

3. Pour into glasses and serve immediately with crushed ice.

Pomegranate Cream

The pomegranate cream is a high-energy drink and should be ideally consumed just before working out or immediately after. It aids in the replenishment of energy in the body and makes you feel refreshed in no time at all! Add in a dash of cayenne for some added spunk to the drink!

Ingredients:

- 2 pears
- 1 large pomegranate
- 2 cups yogurt
- 1/2 cup almond milk

Instructions:

1. Peel the pomegranate and extract the seeds.
2. Core and chop the pears.
3. Juice the pears and pomegranate in a juicer.
4. Add yogurt to a bowl and beat it lightly. Add almond milk and beat again.
5. Pour the juice into it and stir.
6. Pour into individual serving bowls and serve.

Vanilla Yogurt Fruit Smoothie

"Heavenly" is the word you will use to describe the Vanilla Yogurt Fruit Smoothie. With ingredients like pineapples, berries and oranges, this smoothie is high in vitamins and rich in antioxidants. Consume with breakfast and you will have a healthy and glowing skin in no time at all!

Ingredients:

- 1 cup fresh pineapple cubes
- 1 cup raspberries
- 1/2 cup blueberries
- 1/2 cup blackberries
- 4 oranges
- 2 cups low fat vanilla yogurt, unsweetened

Instructions:

1. Peel the oranges and separate into segments.
2. Juice the oranges in a juicer.
3. Add all the ingredients into a blender along with the orange juice. Blend until smooth.
4. Pour into glasses and serve with crushed ice.

Conclusion

Thank you again for choosing this book!

I hope this book was able to help you in understanding the different benefits healthy juices have got to offer. If you are on a diet and you want to lose a couple of inches without depriving your body of essential nutrients, then you can make use of these healthy and tasty juicing recipes for achieving your goal. You will not only be losing weight but you will also be able to make sure that you stay healthy.

The next step is to simply gather all the necessary ingredients and get started with following the recipes to recreate simple and tasty juices that will help you in achieving your health and weight goals. Shopping for the necessary ingredients will not take you long because of the detailed list of ingredients that have been provided in the book along with the recipes. You cannot only follow the recipes that have been mentioned in the book but you can also come up with variation of these recipes. Now that you are equipped with the knowledge regarding the nutritional aspects of various fruits and vegetables, you can experiment and come up with different delicious juices and smoothies. The next time you find yourself craving for something sweet or you just feel like indulging in an evening snack, then instead of grabbing a sugary and starchy snack, you can whip up one of the simple juicing recipes given in this book.

Finally, if you enjoyed this book, then I'd like to ask you for a favor, would you be kind enough to leave a review for this book on Amazon? It'd be greatly appreciated!

Thank you and good luck!

www.ingramcontent.com/pod-product-compliance
Lightning Source LLC
Chambersburg PA
CBHW070242290526
45789CB00004B/1735